30 Days of Belief Work: The Jumpstart

Other Books by Allie Duzett:

Deep Past Resolution

The Scribbling Solution

30 Days of Belief Work: The Jumpstart

By Allie Duzett

356 East 1150 South, Springville, UT 84663
240.316.7389

Cover art created by Mandi Felici

By accepting this book the participant understands that it is not intended to be used as a sole source of mental or physical health care. While all attempts have been made to verify the information provided in this class and workbook, neither Allie Duzett nor Duzett Consulting LLC assumes any responsibility for errors or contradictory interpretations of information contained herein. Acceptance or usage of this book implies full knowledge of all liabilities as expressly disclaimed. Any perceived reference to specific persons or organizations is unintentional. In situations where it is appropriate, it is suggested that all readers consult their own mental health care provider prior to engaging in the exercises herein.

Foreword

Scientists estimate that from the moment we are born to about age 7 or 8 we are forming a majority of our beliefs about the world and how it works. These beliefs will shape our whole reality, our sense of self and how we show up in our relationships and work. Every person has a unique set of beliefs living in their subconscious mind based on their family environment, the society they live in and their trauma.

Everything starts with a belief. When we have an experience, the beliefs we create based on that experience influences our thoughts about that experience, and those thoughts then create feelings in our bodies, positive or negative. Those feelings then influence how we act, and that determines the outcome of what we experience in our reality.

We can shift our life and our experiences dramatically just by changing those beliefs!

I have been doing energy and mindset work for almost 9 years. I am certified in many modalities and I have served hundreds of clients over the years. In my experience, belief work is the MOST powerful and simple tool I have used in my practice. I hope that gives you a sense of what this book can do for you.

Allie is one of the greatest healers I've ever met. If you are one of her clients no doubt you already know this. If you are new to her work, just know that this book can help you change your life dramatically. Belief work may seem so simple, but I can tell you from my knowledge and experience with what it can do for people that you won't regret doing this work. Use Allie's book just as she has set it up and you will have taken a huge step towards changing your life for the better!

Holly Harris
www.theintuitivemind.org
www.secretsofthesubconscious.com

Introduction

This is a book about **beliefs**. All of us have many thousands of belief systems floating around in our bodies and our spirits. Our subconscious minds are FULL of belief programs, and every belief we carry influences everything about our lives.

Our beliefs influence us in two ways.

First, and most obviously, our beliefs color the way we perceive reality. If a person has a belief like "only bad things happen to me," then of course it will be no surprise when they easily notice every bad thing that happens to them—and perhaps completely overlook it when good things happen to them. You might remember this concept this way: **what we perceive, we receive,** and our perceptions are based on our beliefs.

Second, and less obviously, our subconscious beliefs are always projecting out into the world and influencing how the world will react to us. In other words, our life experiences are essentially the world's reaction to our inner belief system. When our inner belief system is "buggy," when it is full of negativity, the outer world reacts to that. The outer world presents back to us what is going on in the inner depths of our souls.

Yes: this does mean that to some extent, if your life has been terrible, it has had something to do with your own internal belief systems.

I understand this is a triggering concept. It is much more comfortable and comforting to say: it's not your fault you were victimized, poor you, nothing is fair in this world. However, Reality as I understand it is predicated on **agency:** our *choices* interacting with and even creating our external circumstances. The big problem is that much of our choices are actually *sub*conscious. This means that while your mind might not consciously be embracing self-sabotage, below the surface, you might still be.

A 2008 study from scientists from the Max Planck Institute for Human Cognitive and Brain Sciences in Leipzig, in collaboration with the Charité University Hospital and the Bernstein Center for Computational Neuroscience in Berlin, found that researchers could predict a person's choice up to *seven seconds in advance* just by looking at the participant's brain before they made a decision. In other words, your brain knows what decisions you will make before your consciousness does.

Your brain is a physical organ, the place where your beliefs are formed. This is where *neural pathways* are constructed and operated. Neural pathways are essentially our beliefs themselves, as physical structures within our brains. When we change how we think, we change our neural pathways: we literally change our brains.

This is why belief work is so important. This is why it is *critical* to bridge the gap between the conscious and subconscious minds, and start finding the unhelpful beliefs and replacing them with helpful ones. If our brains make our decisions before we do, we owe it to ourselves to do what we can to help our brains make the best decisions they can make for us.

And this is what this book is all about: changing the belief systems within us so that we can experience good instead of bad. It's about digging into the brain itself so we can alter both our perception of reality and our *experience* of reality.

It's about giving ourselves our best chance at a happy, successful life.

When I first started my healing journey with belief work, I learned complicated techniques that took a lot of work, and I wasn't always sure they were effective. I would sit on the floor in my bedroom closet, so my skeptical husband couldn't see me, and I would work through these complex exercises every night… and then I would wonder if they had made any difference at all.

I tell you this because as you work through this book, you may not always feel radically different. And that is okay, and that is normal. The point is to just keep going. Just keep doing the exercises. Don't plan on seeing massive changes immediately. Your goal is not immediate massive shifts. Your goal is based on the principle of **compound interest**.

The law of compound interest means that as you put forth just a little bit of effort every single day, over time that effort compounds and compounds and compounds and creates incredible leverage for you. It's the regular effort plus time, added together, that starts making the difference.

For me, I didn't notice immense changes in myself right away when I started doing daily belief work. But over time, it did add up. Weeks into my journey, I realized: "Hey, I'm thinking differently!" And, "Hey, I'm acting differently!"

And that's what it's all about. You don't have to believe your efforts are working; just putting forth the effort over time counts.

There was a time in my life when I felt completely consumed by my own traumas. Everything in my life was hard: my health, my marriage, my job, my finances... literally all of my relationships. But as I healed up my troublesome belief programming, my life got easier and easier. Now I feel like the hardest part of my life is just navigating my business, and my business is trying to make information like this available to as many people as possible!

I feel like now my problems are great problems to have. I love waking up in the morning and having my life overflowing with positive relationships. My marriage is happy, my kids are happy, my bank account is happy. Of course I still have hard days and I still catch colds and my kids still yell and call each other names and drive me crazy and so on and so forth from time to time, but overall, life is much better than it used to be, and I do believe a solid foundation in belief work has a lot to do with that.

My dream is for everyone to have a fabulous, fun life with happy problems instead of sad problems. We all have problems… but I do believe that we all choose our problems on a subconscious level. *So why not choose problems you enjoy solving?*

In order to realize my dream of everyone having happy problems, I do a lot of group energy healing work as part of my business, and I love that aspect of my work. You can check out my group sessions at allieduzettclasses.com. I love making life-changing energy work available to everyone who wants it.

But I will tell you my deepest truth. My biggest motivation is *pain*. I am a Christian—although you do *not* need to be a Christian to benefit from my work—and every day I think of Jesus on the cross and His admonition in Matthew 25:40: "Inasmuch as ye have done it unto the least of these my brethren, ye have done it unto me." I am on a quest to reduce the amount of total pain in this world, and I do it because I am crazy about Jesus. I serve others because I love Him. And this love motivates me to try and figure out new ways, faster ways, to help more people heal more and more quickly.

So I love my group energy work and my personal sessions, but my goal for this book is a little different. I wanted to create a tool that you could use on your own time to start really making serious progress on your own. I want this book to be helpful all on its own, I want it to be helpful as a springboard into greater healing, and I want it to be helpful in combination with my other available work.

I hope it blesses not just you, but also your children, your spouse, your ancestors, and everyone you know. Because as *you* change, **you will change the world for everyone who ever interacts with you.**

So let's get to work changing and healing our brains. You might not feel totally different right away, and that's okay. All I ask is that you just keep going! Keep working at it for at least a few consecutive weeks before really assessing the changes you've experienced and noticed within yourself. This work can very seriously change your life for the better, and that is my ultimate goal.

Take the 30-Day Belief Work Pledge

I, ______________________________, hereby commit to completing at least 30 consecutive days of belief work and assessing the difference I feel within.

Signature: ______________________________

How This Book Works

I've designed this book to help you get started on your belief work journey. If you've already started doing belief work in the past, my goal is to help you jumpstart and supercharge that process. I've chosen a number of very common destructive beliefs to remove from our systems every day. In their place, you'll "download" powerful positive replacements.

Before I explain how shifting beliefs works, I want to teach you a technique you can use to have greater insight into your body and mind. Mastering this tool will help you make more progress, faster.

Tuning In With Your Body

One technique I love to teach my students is called "intuitive calibration." If you go to the Allie Duzett YouTube channel, you can watch a video about it, but it's very simple to explain.

ife in this mortal plane is a series of breaths. The ancients understood that life and breath and spirit are all just aspects of the same thing.

The Greek word *pneuma* means both "soul" and "breath." The Latin *anima spiritus* means both "spirit" and "breath." The Hebrew word for breath is the same exact word as is used for "Spirit of God." To "inspire" literally means to "breathe in," so there may be some application to the idea that if you are having trouble feeling the Holy Spirit, maybe you need to breathe more deeply to get *inspired.* There is an ancient understanding that the spirit and the breath are uniquely, deeply connected.

The breath is miraculous because it is one of two automatic bodily processes that can be controlled by the conscious mind--the other, incidentally, is blinking, which is also rich in symbolism and in application. Because of this unique aspect of breath--being a process that is both conscious and subconscious--we can actually use the breath to access the subconscious mind.

Understanding the subconscious mind is deeply important to living in alignment with ourselves and to unlocking our hidden gifts and potential. How many of us have had an experience where, in the moment, we knew what we were doing was wrong, but it just came to us so second-nature that we couldn't stop it? Those moments are run by the subconscious mind. And even though we may not have felt in control of ourselves in those moments, the things we do and the bad choices we make under the influence of the subconscious mind are still things we are accountable for and things we need to change.

Yogi Bhajan, the Mahan Tantric of Kundalini Yoga who introduced this form of yoga to the United States in the 1960's, taught that most people breathe too shallowly to maintain even normal health. So as you focus on your breathing this week and in the future, you will notice a shift in both your physical and mental health.

You start your own intuitive calibration by taking deep breaths and closing your eyes. After a few deep breaths, you ask your body: "Body, what does a 'yes' feel like?" And you just breathe and breathe and see what it feels like in your body.

When I asked one class of students to describe how they felt when asking their bodies to show them a "yes" feeling, this is what they came up with:

- feelings of light or warmth or tingling in the lungs and face
- feelings of spiritual expansion
- feelings of energy rising in the body
- feelings of spiritual "smiling"
- open feelings in the heart area

After you spend a few minutes feeling what a "yes" feels like in *your* body, shake yourself out, and try again. This time, though, you ask: "Body, what does a 'no' feel like?" And breathe and breathe again, so deeply, and see what a "no" feels like in your body.

When I asked that same group of students to describe a "no" feeling, they came up with this list:

- feelings of being closed off
- energy sinking downward instead of upward
- tingling on different parts of the body (one person's guts sometimes tingle when their body is telling them no, and another person's ears tingle)
- feelings of constriction

Each body responds differently and communicates the answers to these questions in different ways, but there seems to be some commonalities across the board.

One other thing I like to have my students check for is how their bodies will present a "false yes" or a "false no." They report that when they ask their bodies to show them what false answers feel like, they typically feel dizziness, movement in their bodies that is not the same as a "yes" or "no," or tingling in different parts of their body than they experience with a true "yes" or a true "no."

With this process of intuitive calibration, you can have a baseline for understanding how your own body communicates with you, and if your body is trying to give you a "false yes" or a "false no," you will also know how to spot that. You could also ask your body to show you how it feels when your body is trying to confuse you.

In case you are wondering why a body might try to confuse its owner, sometimes our bodies or subconscious minds try to confuse our conscious selves because they think it will keep us safe. The primary function of both the body and the subconscious mind is to keep us as safe as possible. Sometimes new concepts make the subconscious mind uncomfortable because they may prompt changes that seem unsafe. If or when this happens, the subconscious mind can respond to these concepts with confusion designed to prevent us from making changes that seem scary.

But when you put in the time and work to truly get acquainted with your body's responses to "yes" and "no," it can simplify your life enormously.

If you are a praying person, you can use this technique in combination with prayer. You do this asking in prayer for God to show you through your own body's feelings and sensations how He communicates with you the ideas of "yes" and "no" (and "maybe"--which is sometimes an answer as well!).

If you are not a praying person, you can use this as an easy way to immediately discern your own soul's feelings about a situation, right there, in the moment.

Either way, this is a simple but profound technique for getting more in tune with your own self and living more fully in a space of true integrity to your own soul.

I urge you to try this technique before reading any further. One beautiful thing about life is that it is a series of breaths, which means that once you master this technique, you can feel it instantly any time anything is in alignment with you, or if it isn't.

As you read this book, I invite you to do it with your breath in mind--or, should I say, with your breath in heart. I invite you to use your breath and your body to help you feel out what is resonant with you.

Using Intuitive Calibration With Belief Work

Intuitive calibration is very helpful with belief work, because it provides another form of feedback for you to use in making your assessments of your own belief journey.

What I mean by this is that you can use intuitive calibration to help you decide *what* beliefs you really need to address, *how* to address them, and to assess afterwards if the issue has been fully resolved or not.

Once you learn your own body's responses to "yes" and "no," you can ask yourself all sorts of questions that can help you on your journey through this world.

When it comes to belief work, intuitive calibration is the technique you can use to ask yourself:

- Is this belief fully dissolved and resolved?
- Is there another related belief program I should work on pertaining to this issue?
- Am I missing something here?

This is a great technique for gaining clarity on whatever you are working on in your life. Ask yourself plenty of thoughtful "yes" and "no" questions to help yourself discern with clarity what belief you need to be working on next and how to work on it.

his is something you can practice right now. As you master intuitive calibration, you will find that you can receive answers about anything you want or need, just by living your daily life. Just being consciously aware of your breath and your body will give you so much more information than you ever realized was possible.

How To Do Belief Work

There are lots of ways to do belief work. Many books and programs already exist to help people do this kind of work. What I have curated here is a *simplified* version of the work that I hope will make this accessible and simple for everyday people who may not be familiar with the ins and outs of fancier energy work systems.

So this is how my system works for the purposes of this book, the step-by-step process.

1. Tap on your forehead, knees, *or* collarbone while repeating aloud the belief you need to release. You may need to repeat the belief aloud several times.

2. Imagine the old belief written out on a ribbon in your brain. As you tap and speak the belief, imagine the ribbon being sucked out of your head, completely removed.

3. Take a deep breath.

4. Replace the old belief with a new belief by imagining the words of the new belief on a new, clean, bright ribbon.

5. Tap on your forehead, knees, or collarbone while repeating the words of the new belief.

6. Imagine the new belief ribbon threading into your brain and body and spirit. Imagine it wrapping around and in and through all of your individual cells.

7. When you are done, take a deep breath and imagine your own cells and your own spirit giving you a thumbs up.

Some notes on this process:

- If you can't imagine a "thumbs up" at the end, it means something went wrong and perhaps the belief you were working to replace was too thoroughly ingrained to leave easily. If that is the case, please try "scribbling" on the belief (see the appendix for instructions).

- You actually *don't* need to say the words out loud for the process to work. You also don't need to tap. But those are helpful in the beginning, while you are getting used to the mental process of doing the work. I recommend doing the tapping and the speaking aloud in the beginning, because the physical cues can help strengthen the habit and help you feel the changes more thoroughly in your physical body. When you feel like a practiced master at this style of belief work, you can do the work mentally alone, just by imagining the ribbons.

Doing Belief Work By Proxy

I recommend doing the belief work for yourself first, but after you have done it for yourself, it is possible to do the belief work by proxy, for your children and those in your legal guardianship. When doing belief work for a child, do the tapping and speaking yourself, but imagine that it is taking place on behalf of the child. When you are imagining an old belief getting released, imagine it releasing from that child. When you imagine the replacement, imagine it getting replaced in the child's energy field. It is very simple to do! But please work on yourself first. You are your own top priority.

I do not recommend doing this work for spouses, even if they give permission, because I feel strongly that when a spouse is not interested in this work, it is most appropriate to give them their space, and not try to change them. If a spouse notices the amazing changes you are experiencing and wants to know more about why, that's when you would hand them a copy of this book and invite them to give it a try.

I believe doing belief work by proxy for minors in your legal guardianship is okay, but for those over the age of 18 who are physically capable of doing this work themselves, it is best to let them do it for themselves.

When we start trying to save everyone we know by doing belief work for them, we are exhibiting bad boundaries and we are robbing our loved ones of the opportunity to take responsibility for their own lives.

It is not your job to save anyone else. YOU are your primary responsibility in life. Just changing yourself will lead to powerful changes in everyone around you. You don't need to go crazy trying to fix everyone around you as well.

Getting Started

As you work through this book, every day you will be presented with a handful of beliefs to work through, on a variety of different topics. The idea is that you will just work on that day's set of beliefs, and not skip ahead or jump around. The goal is that you will not be overwhelmed, you will not burn yourself out; you will just make slow and steady progress every day, and over time you will look back and see how different things are—in a very positive way!

I recommend doing these beliefs in the order I curated them. I put them in that order because they build on each other and support each other.

At the same time, I definitely honor each person's intuition above all. So if your intuition is telling you to flip open to a random page and work through beliefs there also, then by golly, I guess you should listen to your own intuition on that.

If a belief is very triggering for you, I do recommend flipping to the section on scribbling at the back of the book. This is the tool you will use to get out of trigger mode and solidly into healing mode. Follow the instructions there to scribble out your triggers, and *then* do the belief work. You will see major shifts after clearing things that were previously triggering!

This is an introductory belief work book, one with a wide variety of beliefs to work through. You'll find belief work around anger, sorrow, irritation, betrayal, and more. My goal is for this book to work as a sort of "jumpstart" to target a number of important areas of *your* life, so that you can experience positive shifts in well-being in many areas of your life over the course of the thirty days.

With no further ado, please turn the page and get started with Day 1! I am so thrilled and excited for you to start seeing some shifts as you begin doing this important healing work!

DAY 1

Way to get started! Today we're clearing beliefs on **worthiness**. Feel free to write any thoughts you have about your experiences in the margins, or use the white space on this page to scribble out any emotions that come up as you do your tapping, removal, and replacement.

As a reminder: Tap while repeating aloud the belief you need to release. You may need to repeat the belief aloud several times. Imagine the old belief written out on a ribbon in your brain. As you tap and speak the belief, imagine the ribbon being sucked out of your head. Replace the old belief with a new belief by imagining the words of the new belief on a new, clean, bright ribbon. Tap while repeating the words of the new belief. Imagine the new belief ribbon threading into your brain and body and spirit. Imagine it wrapping around and in and through all of your individual cells. When you are done, take a deep breath and imagine your own cells and your own spirit giving you a thumbs up.

Remove:

- I don't deserve to heal.
- I can't change my beliefs.
- I am unworthy of having a good life.
- I deserve a bad life.
- I deserve to be sad.

Replace with:

- I deserve to heal.

- I can change my beliefs.
- I am worthy of having a good life.
- I deserve a happy life.
- I deserve to be glad every day that I am alive.

Scribbling Page

Scribbling Page

DAY 2

Way to get started! Today we're continuing to clear beliefs on **worthiness**. Feel free to write any thoughts you have about your experiences in the margins, or use the white space on this page to scribble out any emotions that come up as you do your tapping, removal, and replacement.

As a reminder: Tap while repeating aloud the belief you need to release. You may need to repeat the belief aloud several times. Imagine the old belief written out on a ribbon in your brain. As you tap and speak the belief, imagine the ribbon being sucked out of your head. Replace the old belief with a new belief by imagining the words of the new belief on a new, clean, bright ribbon. Tap while repeating the words of the new belief. Imagine the new belief ribbon threading into your brain and body and spirit. Imagine it wrapping around and in and through all of your individual cells. When you are done, take a deep breath and imagine your own cells and your own spirit giving you a thumbs up.

Remove:

- I am not worthy of money.
- I am not worthy of a loving relationship.
- I am unworthy.
- I cannot have the things I want.
- I deserve heartbreak and trauma.

Replace with:

- I deserve to have all the money I need!

- I am worthy of a loving, accepting relationship.
- I am WORTHY of GOOD THINGS!
- I CAN have the things I want!
- I deserve joy and peace every day of my life.

Scribbling Page

Scribbling Page

DAY 3

Today we're clearing beliefs on **shame**. Feel free to write any thoughts you have about your experiences in the margins, or use the white space on this page to scribble out any emotions that come up as you do your tapping, removal, and replacement.

As a reminder: Tap while repeating aloud the belief you need to release. You may need to repeat the belief aloud several times. Imagine the old belief written out on a ribbon in your brain. As you tap and speak the belief, imagine the ribbon being sucked out of your head. Replace the old belief with a new belief by imagining the words of the new belief on a new, clean, bright ribbon. Tap while repeating the words of the new belief. Imagine the new belief ribbon threading into your brain and body and spirit. Imagine it wrapping around and in and through all of your individual cells. When you are done, take a deep breath and imagine your own cells and your own spirit giving you a thumbs up.

Remove:

- I am ashamed.
- My existence is shameful.
- I am embarrassed to exist.
- I should be ashamed of myself.
- I should be ashamed of my past.

Replace with:

- I know how to live life without feeling shame.

- My existence is beautiful and important.
- I deserve to exist.
- I deserve to exist in joy and self-acceptance.
- I know how to live life accepting myself.
- I know how to live life feeling peace about my past and where I came from.

Scribbling Page

Scribbling Page

DAY 4

Today we're clearing beliefs on **fear**. Feel free to write any thoughts you have about your experiences in the margins, or use the white space on this page to scribble out any emotions that come up as you do your tapping, removal, and replacement.

As a reminder: Tap while repeating aloud the belief you need to release. You may need to repeat the belief aloud several times. Imagine the old belief written out on a ribbon in your brain. As you tap and speak the belief, imagine the ribbon being sucked out of your head. Replace the old belief with a new belief by imagining the words of the new belief on a new, clean, bright ribbon. Tap while repeating the words of the new belief. Imagine the new belief ribbon threading into your brain and body and spirit. Imagine it wrapping around and in and through all of your individual cells. When you are done, take a deep breath and imagine your own cells and your own spirit giving you a thumbs up.

Remove:

- I am afraid.
- Fear is important to my safety.
- I don't know how to live without fear.
- I have to be afraid to survive.
- Good people are afraid.

Replace with:

- I know how to live without fear.

- I know how to live with courage.
- I have a courageous heart.
- Courage is the most important thing to my safety.
- Good people have courage.

Scribbling Page

Scribbling Page

DAY 5

Today we're continuing to clear beliefs on **fear**. Feel free to write any thoughts you have about your experiences in the margins, or use the white space on this page to scribble out any emotions that come up as you do your tapping, removal, and replacement.

As a reminder: Tap while repeating aloud the belief you need to release. You may need to repeat the belief aloud several times. Imagine the old belief written out on a ribbon in your brain. As you tap and speak the belief, imagine the ribbon being sucked out of your head. Replace the old belief with a new belief by imagining the words of the new belief on a new, clean, bright ribbon. Tap while repeating the words of the new belief. Imagine the new belief ribbon threading into your brain and body and spirit. Imagine it wrapping around and in and through all of your individual cells. When you are done, take a deep breath and imagine your own cells and your own spirit giving you a thumbs up.

Remove:

- I am afraid of other people.
- I am afraid of my mother.
- I am afraid of my father.
- I am afraid of God.
- I am afraid of being judged.

Replace with:

- I know how to live without fear of other people.

- I know how to live without fear of my mother.
- I know how to live without fear of my father.
- I know how to live without fear of God.
- I know how to live without fear of being judged.

Scribbling Page

Scribbling Page

DAY 6

Today we're continuing to clear beliefs on **fear**. Feel free to write any thoughts you have about your experiences in the margins, or use the white space on this page to scribble out any emotions that come up as you do your tapping, removal, and replacement.

As a reminder: Tap while repeating aloud the belief you need to release. You may need to repeat the belief aloud several times. Imagine the old belief written out on a ribbon in your brain. As you tap and speak the belief, imagine the ribbon being sucked out of your head. Replace the old belief with a new belief by imagining the words of the new belief on a new, clean, bright ribbon. Tap while repeating the words of the new belief. Imagine the new belief ribbon threading into your brain and body and spirit. Imagine it wrapping around and in and through all of your individual cells. When you are done, take a deep breath and imagine your own cells and your own spirit giving you a thumbs up.

Remove:

- I am afraid of sharing who I am.
- I am afraid of my fertility.
- I am afraid of my body.
- I am afraid of being fat.
- I am afraid of being thin.

Replace with:

- I know how to live without fear of sharing who I am.

- It is safe for me to share who I am.
- I know how to live without fearing my fertility.
- I feel safe when I think about my fertility.
- I know how to live without fear of my body.
- I feel safe inside my body.
- I know how to live without fear of being fat.
- I love myself and all the fat on my body.
- I know how to live without fear of being thin.
- I love myself without fear of being thin.

Scribbling Page

Scribbling Page

DAY 7

Today we're continuing to clear beliefs on **fear**. Feel free to write any thoughts you have about your experiences in the margins, or use the white space on this page to scribble out any emotions that come up as you do your tapping, removal, and replacement.

As a reminder: Tap while repeating aloud the belief you need to release. You may need to repeat the belief aloud several times. Imagine the old belief written out on a ribbon in your brain. As you tap and speak the belief, imagine the ribbon being sucked out of your head. Replace the old belief with a new belief by imagining the words of the new belief on a new, clean, bright ribbon. Tap while repeating the words of the new belief. Imagine the new belief ribbon threading into your brain and body and spirit. Imagine it wrapping around and in and through all of your individual cells. When you are done, take a deep breath and imagine your own cells and your own spirit giving you a thumbs up.

Remove:

- I am afraid of being honest.
- I am afraid of sharing my truth.
- I am afraid of being myself.
- I am afraid of what others think of me.
- I am afraid of getting in trouble.

Replace with:

- It is safe for me to be honest.

- I can share my truth fearlessly.
- I feel safe being myself.
- I know how to live feeling love for myself no matter what others think of me.
- I know how to live without fearing getting in trouble.

Scribbling Page

Scribbling Page

DAY 8

Today we're clearing more beliefs on **shame.** Feel free to write any thoughts you have about your experiences in the margins, or use the white space on this page to scribble out any emotions that come up as you do your tapping, removal, and replacement.

As a reminder: Tap while repeating aloud the belief you need to release. You may need to repeat the belief aloud several times. Imagine the old belief written out on a ribbon in your brain. As you tap and speak the belief, imagine the ribbon being sucked out of your head. Replace the old belief with a new belief by imagining the words of the new belief on a new, clean, bright ribbon. Tap while repeating the words of the new belief. Imagine the new belief ribbon threading into your brain and body and spirit. Imagine it wrapping around and in and through all of your individual cells. When you are done, take a deep breath and imagine your own cells and your own spirit giving you a thumbs up.

Remove:

- I am ashamed of my body.
- I am ashamed of my finances.
- I am ashamed of the state of my house.
- I am ashamed of being who I am.
- There is something wrong with me.

Replace with:

- I know how to live without shame about my body.

- I choose to love my body exactly as it is in this moment.
- I know how to live without shame about my finances.
- I choose to feel happy and grateful for the role money plays in my life.
- I know how to live without feeling shame about being who I am.
- I love who I am!
- There is nothing wrong with me!
- I am exactly right for this stage of my journey.
- I am exactly the right person at the right place at the right time, for myself.

Scribbling Page

Scribbling Page

DAY 9

Today we're clearing beliefs on **pride**. Feel free to write any thoughts you have about your experiences in the margins, or use the white space on this page to scribble out any emotions that come up as you do your tapping, removal, and replacement.

As a reminder: Tap while repeating aloud the belief you need to release. You may need to repeat the belief aloud several times. Imagine the old belief written out on a ribbon in your brain. As you tap and speak the belief, imagine the ribbon being sucked out of your head. Replace the old belief with a new belief by imagining the words of the new belief on a new, clean, bright ribbon. Tap while repeating the words of the new belief. Imagine the new belief ribbon threading into your brain and body and spirit. Imagine it wrapping around and in and through all of your individual cells. When you are done, take a deep breath and imagine your own cells and your own spirit giving you a thumbs up.

Remove:

- I am better than others.
- I am entitled to respect from others.
- I am more deserving than others.
- I am a better person than other people.
- I am always right.
- I have to be right.

Replace with:

- All men and women are created equal.
- Great is the worth of ALL souls in the eyes of God.
- I know how to live without feeling entitled to more than others.
- I am not the judge of who deserves what.
- I know how to live without feeling better than others.
- I know how to live without feeling like I have to always be right.
- I don't always have to be right.
- It can be safe to be wrong.

Scribbling Page

Scribbling Page

DAY 10

Today we're clearing beliefs on **shock**. Feel free to write any thoughts you have about your experiences in the margins, or use the white space on this page to scribble out any emotions that come up as you do your tapping, removal, and replacement.

As a reminder: Tap while repeating aloud the belief you need to release. You may need to repeat the belief aloud several times. Imagine the old belief written out on a ribbon in your brain. As you tap and speak the belief, imagine the ribbon being sucked out of your head. Replace the old belief with a new belief by imagining the words of the new belief on a new, clean, bright ribbon. Tap while repeating the words of the new belief. Imagine the new belief ribbon threading into your brain and body and spirit. Imagine it wrapping around and in and through all of your individual cells. When you are done, take a deep breath and imagine your own cells and your own spirit giving you a thumbs up.

Remove:

- I am shocked.
- Living in a constant state of shock is important.
- If I'm always shocked, new shocking things cannot surprise me.
- Being chronically shocked helps me stay safe.
- I don't know how to live without shock.

Replace with:

- I know how to live without feeling shock.
- Constant shock is not necessary to a happy life.
- It is safe to allow feelings of shock to run through me.
- I do not need to hold onto chronic feelings of shock.
- It is safe to feel shock when surprising things happen, and then to let the shock drain from me so I can handle the event.

Scribbling Page

Scribbling Page

DAY 11

Today we're clearing beliefs on **betrayal**. Feel free to write any thoughts you have about your experiences in the margins, or use the white space on this page to scribble out any emotions that come up as you do your tapping, removal, and replacement.

As a reminder: Tap while repeating aloud the belief you need to release. You may need to repeat the belief aloud several times. Imagine the old belief written out on a ribbon in your brain. As you tap and speak the belief, imagine the ribbon being sucked out of your head. Replace the old belief with a new belief by imagining the words of the new belief on a new, clean, bright ribbon. Tap while repeating the words of the new belief. Imagine the new belief ribbon threading into your brain and body and spirit. Imagine it wrapping around and in and through all of your individual cells. When you are done, take a deep breath and imagine your own cells and your own spirit giving you a thumbs up.

Remove:

- I am always betrayed.
- Everyone betrays me.
- God has betrayed me.
- Reality betrays me.
- I don't know how to live without being betrayed.

Replace with:

- I know how to live without being betrayed.

- I live free from betrayal.
- I open my heart to God's divine perspective on my perceived betrayals.
- I choose to believe in a loving Universe that works only and always for my greatest good.

Scribbling Page

Scribbling Page

DAY 12

Today we're continuing to clear beliefs on **betrayal.** Feel free to write any thoughts you have about your experiences in the margins, or use the white space on this page to scribble out any emotions that come up as you do your tapping, removal, and replacement.

As a reminder: Tap while repeating aloud the belief you need to release. You may need to repeat the belief aloud several times. Imagine the old belief written out on a ribbon in your brain. As you tap and speak the belief, imagine the ribbon being sucked out of your head. Replace the old belief with a new belief by imagining the words of the new belief on a new, clean, bright ribbon. Tap while repeating the words of the new belief. Imagine the new belief ribbon threading into your brain and body and spirit. Imagine it wrapping around and in and through all of your individual cells. When you are done, take a deep breath and imagine your own cells and your own spirit giving you a thumbs up.

Remove:

- I have betrayed myself.
- I am my own greatest betrayer.
- I betray people I care about.
- My body betrays me.
- My emotions betray me.

Replace with:

- I know how to live without feeling like I betray myself.

- I am doing the best I can.
- I choose to forgive myself for the times I have acted as a betrayer.
- I forgive my body for perceived betrayals.
- I love my body.
- I accept my emotions as they are.
- I know my emotions would never intentionally betray me.

Scribbling Page

Scribbling Page

DAY 13

Today we're clearing beliefs on **anger**. Feel free to write any thoughts you have about your experiences in the margins, or use the white space on this page to scribble out any emotions that come up as you do your tapping, removal, and replacement.

As a reminder: Tap while repeating aloud the belief you need to release. You may need to repeat the belief aloud several times. Imagine the old belief written out on a ribbon in your brain. As you tap and speak the belief, imagine the ribbon being sucked out of your head. Replace the old belief with a new belief by imagining the words of the new belief on a new, clean, bright ribbon. Tap while repeating the words of the new belief. Imagine the new belief ribbon threading into your brain and body and spirit. Imagine it wrapping around and in and through all of your individual cells. When you are done, take a deep breath and imagine your own cells and your own spirit giving you a thumbs up.

Remove:

- I deserve to feel angry.
- Anger is an important emotion to feel every day.
- Anger makes me feel alive.
- Anger makes me feel validated.
- I am safer when I am angry.
- People respect me more when I am angry.

Replace with:

- I know how to live without feeling anger.
- I choose to live life free from chronic anger.
- I know how to feel alive without feeling angry.
- I am safest when I keep a clear mind and heart.
- People respect me most when I am calm.
- I know how to feel validated without turning to anger.

Scribbling Page

Scribbling Page

DAY 14

Today we're clearing beliefs on **irritation**. Feel free to write any thoughts you have about your experiences in the margins, or use the white space on this page to scribble out any emotions that come up as you do your tapping, removal, and replacement.

As a reminder: Tap while repeating aloud the belief you need to release. You may need to repeat the belief aloud several times. Imagine the old belief written out on a ribbon in your brain. As you tap and speak the belief, imagine the ribbon being sucked out of your head. Replace the old belief with a new belief by imagining the words of the new belief on a new, clean, bright ribbon. Tap while repeating the words of the new belief. Imagine the new belief ribbon threading into your brain and body and spirit. Imagine it wrapping around and in and through all of your individual cells. When you are done, take a deep breath and imagine your own cells and your own spirit giving you a thumbs up.

Remove:

- I deserve to feel irritated.
- Other people are irritating.
- I irritate myself.
- People who are different from me are irritating.
- All my irritation with others is justified.
- All my irritation with myself is justified.

Replace with:

- I know how to live without feeling irritated with others.
- I know how to live without feeling irritated by myself.
- I deserve to feel at peace with other people's choices.
- I know how to love and accept those who are different from me, even if I previously have found them irritating.
- My enormous sense of peace with the decisions and actions of others is justified.

Scribbling Page

Scribbling Page

DAY 15

Today we're continuing to clear beliefs on **irritation**. Feel free to write any thoughts you have about your experiences in the margins, or use the white space on this page to scribble out any emotions that come up as you do your tapping, removal, and replacement.

As a reminder: Tap while repeating aloud the belief you need to release. You may need to repeat the belief aloud several times. Imagine the old belief written out on a ribbon in your brain. As you tap and speak the belief, imagine the ribbon being sucked out of your head. Replace the old belief with a new belief by imagining the words of the new belief on a new, clean, bright ribbon. Tap while repeating the words of the new belief. Imagine the new belief ribbon threading into your brain and body and spirit. Imagine it wrapping around and in and through all of your individual cells. When you are done, take a deep breath and imagine your own cells and your own spirit giving you a thumbs up.

Remove:

- My body is in a constant state of irritation.
- I don't know how to live without internal irritation and inflammation.
- Internal irritation is important to the function of my body.
- My immune system doesn't know how to handle its irritations.
- Body-level irritation is important to me.

Replace with:

- I know how to let go of my fear of living without irritation.
- It is safe for me to live without irritation.
- It is safe for me to live without body-level irritation.
- My immune system has God's divine perspective on how to handle the things that irritate it, safely and effectively.
- My body functions better and better as it decreases its body-level irritations.

Scribbling Page

Scribbling Page

DAY 16

Today we're continuing to clear beliefs on **irritation**. Feel free to write any thoughts you have about your experiences in the margins, or use the white space on this page to scribble out any emotions that come up as you do your tapping, removal, and replacement.

As a reminder: Tap while repeating aloud the belief you need to release. You may need to repeat the belief aloud several times. Imagine the old belief written out on a ribbon in your brain. As you tap and speak the belief, imagine the ribbon being sucked out of your head. Replace the old belief with a new belief by imagining the words of the new belief on a new, clean, bright ribbon. Tap while repeating the words of the new belief. Imagine the new belief ribbon threading into your brain and body and spirit. Imagine it wrapping around and in and through all of your individual cells. When you are done, take a deep breath and imagine your own cells and your own spirit giving you a thumbs up.

Remove:

- My relatives irritate me.
- My mother irritates me.
- My father irritates me.
- My siblings irritate me.
- My life circumstances irritate me.

Replace with:

- I know how to live without feeling irritation at my relatives.
- I know how to live without feeling irritation at my mother.
- I know how to live without feeling irritation at my father.
- I know how to live without feeling irritation at my siblings.
- I know how to live without feeling irritation at my life circumstances.
- I know my life circumstances are exactly right for me at this time.
- As I uplevel my belief programming and my emotional healing, my life circumstances will heal and change to reflect my internal work in a positive way.

Scribbling Page

Scribbling Page

DAY 17

Today we're continuing to clear beliefs on **irritation**. Feel free to write any thoughts you have about your experiences in the margins, or use the white space on this page to scribble out any emotions that come up as you do your tapping, removal, and replacement.

As a reminder: Tap while repeating aloud the belief you need to release. You may need to repeat the belief aloud several times. Imagine the old belief written out on a ribbon in your brain. As you tap and speak the belief, imagine the ribbon being sucked out of your head. Replace the old belief with a new belief by imagining the words of the new belief on a new, clean, bright ribbon. Tap while repeating the words of the new belief. Imagine the new belief ribbon threading into your brain and body and spirit. Imagine it wrapping around and in and through all of your individual cells. When you are done, take a deep breath and imagine your own cells and your own spirit giving you a thumbs up.

Remove:

- I am irritated with money.
- Finances irritate me.
- Chores irritate me.
- Working irritates me.
- I feel irritated when I am interrupted.

Replace with:

- I know how to live without feeling irritated with money.
- Finances delight me and comfort me.
- I know how to enjoy my chores.
- I choose to enjoy my chores.
- I choose to enjoy working.
- I enjoy the benefits of my work.
- I know how to experience interruptions without feeling irritated.
- I choose to feel calm and peace even when I am interrupted.

Scribbling Page

Scribbling Page

DAY 18

Today we're clearing beliefs around **confusion**. Feel free to write any thoughts you have about your experiences in the margins, or use the white space on this page to scribble out any emotions that come up as you do your tapping, removal, and replacement.

As a reminder: Tap while repeating aloud the belief you need to release. You may need to repeat the belief aloud several times. Imagine the old belief written out on a ribbon in your brain. As you tap and speak the belief, imagine the ribbon being sucked out of your head. Replace the old belief with a new belief by imagining the words of the new belief on a new, clean, bright ribbon. Tap while repeating the words of the new belief. Imagine the new belief ribbon threading into your brain and body and spirit. Imagine it wrapping around and in and through all of your individual cells. When you are done, take a deep breath and imagine your own cells and your own spirit giving you a thumbs up.

Remove:

- I don't know what I'm doing in life.
- I'm not sure why I'm here.
- What is the point?
- I feel apathetic.
- I don't know what to do next.

Replace with:

- I know what to do next in my life.

- On a body and soul level I know why I am here on the earth.
- I am choosing to open my consciousness to consciously remembering why I am here on this earth.
- I know how to live feeling excitement to be alive.
- I have a constant knowingness of what to do next in my life.
- I feel certain I have a divine mission.

Scribbling Page

Scribbling Page

DAY 19

Today we're working on beliefs around **feeling lost**. Feel free to write any thoughts you have about your experiences in the margins, or use the white space on this page to scribble out any emotions that come up as you do your tapping, removal, and replacement.

As a reminder: Tap while repeating aloud the belief you need to release. You may need to repeat the belief aloud several times. Imagine the old belief written out on a ribbon in your brain. As you tap and speak the belief, imagine the ribbon being sucked out of your head. Replace the old belief with a new belief by imagining the words of the new belief on a new, clean, bright ribbon. Tap while repeating the words of the new belief. Imagine the new belief ribbon threading into your brain and body and spirit. Imagine it wrapping around and in and through all of your individual cells. When you are done, take a deep breath and imagine your own cells and your own spirit giving you a thumbs up.

Remove:

- I feel lost.
- No one cares enough to find me.
- I don't know how to find my way.
- I forgot how to feel a sense of direction.
- I have no sense of direction.

Replace with:

- I have a sense of direction.

- I am moving forward in life.
- I feel "found" and safe.
- I know God is always seeking me.
- I am never lost to God.
- I remember now how to find my way.
- I choose to listen to my own heart and soul to lead my way forward.

Scribbling Page

Scribbling Page

DAY 20

Today we're working on beliefs surrounding **heartbreak**. Feel free to write any thoughts you have about your experiences in the margins, or use the white space on this page to scribble out any emotions that come up as you do your tapping, removal, and replacement.

As a reminder: Tap while repeating aloud the belief you need to release. You may need to repeat the belief aloud several times. Imagine the old belief written out on a ribbon in your brain. As you tap and speak the belief, imagine the ribbon being sucked out of your head. Replace the old belief with a new belief by imagining the words of the new belief on a new, clean, bright ribbon. Tap while repeating the words of the new belief. Imagine the new belief ribbon threading into your brain and body and spirit. Imagine it wrapping around and in and through all of your individual cells. When you are done, take a deep breath and imagine your own cells and your own spirit giving you a thumbs up.

Remove:

- My heart is broken.
- I don't know how to live without heartbreak.
- Heartbreak shows that things are important to me.
- Responsible people feel heartbroken about important things.
- If I heal from heartbreak it means I didn't really care.

Replace with:

- I know how to live without heartbreak.
- I can heal my heartbreak while honoring the situation that broke my heart.
- My heart is healing and healed.
- I know how to care about things without feeling heartbreak over them.
- It is responsible to care about things and love things without experiencing constant heartbreak.

Scribbling Page

Scribbling Page

DAY 21

Today we're working on beliefs around **bodies**. Feel free to write any thoughts you have about your experiences in the margins, or use the white space on this page to scribble out any emotions that come up as you do your tapping, removal, and replacement.

As a reminder: Tap while repeating aloud the belief you need to release. You may need to repeat the belief aloud several times. Imagine the old belief written out on a ribbon in your brain. As you tap and speak the belief, imagine the ribbon being sucked out of your head. Replace the old belief with a new belief by imagining the words of the new belief on a new, clean, bright ribbon. Tap while repeating the words of the new belief. Imagine the new belief ribbon threading into your brain and body and spirit. Imagine it wrapping around and in and through all of your individual cells. When you are done, take a deep breath and imagine your own cells and your own spirit giving you a thumbs up.

Remove:

- I hate my body.
- My body isn't good enough.
- I regret having this body.
- This body was a mistake.
- My body deserves bad things.

Replace with:

- I know how to love my body.

- I choose to love my body.
- I love my body.
- My body is always good enough.
- I love having this body.
- My body is a perfect gift.
- My body deserves the best things.

Scribbling Page

Scribbling Page

DAY 22

Today we're working on beliefs around **romance**. Feel free to write any thoughts you have about your experiences in the margins, or use the white space on this page to scribble out any emotions that come up as you do your tapping, removal, and replacement.

As a reminder: Tap while repeating aloud the belief you need to release. You may need to repeat the belief aloud several times. Imagine the old belief written out on a ribbon in your brain. As you tap and speak the belief, imagine the ribbon being sucked out of your head. Replace the old belief with a new belief by imagining the words of the new belief on a new, clean, bright ribbon. Tap while repeating the words of the new belief. Imagine the new belief ribbon threading into your brain and body and spirit. Imagine it wrapping around and in and through all of your individual cells. When you are done, take a deep breath and imagine your own cells and your own spirit giving you a thumbs up.

Remove:

- Romance is not safe for me.
- I am not good enough for romance.
- Romance is a lie.
- No one could ever love me romantically.
- I do not deserve true love.

Replace with:

- Romance can be safe for me.

- I deserve true love.
- I am good enough for romance and true love.
- I have God's divine definition of true love.
- I know romance can be real and can be truly motivated by pure acceptance and adoration of another person.
- There is someone out there romantically for me.

Scribbling Page

Scribbling Page

DAY 23

Today we're working on beliefs around **pain**. Feel free to write any thoughts you have about your experiences in the margins, or use the white space on this page to scribble out any emotions that come up as you do your tapping, removal, and replacement.

As a reminder: Tap while repeating aloud the belief you need to release. You may need to repeat the belief aloud several times. Imagine the old belief written out on a ribbon in your brain. As you tap and speak the belief, imagine the ribbon being sucked out of your head. Replace the old belief with a new belief by imagining the words of the new belief on a new, clean, bright ribbon. Tap while repeating the words of the new belief. Imagine the new belief ribbon threading into your brain and body and spirit. Imagine it wrapping around and in and through all of your individual cells. When you are done, take a deep breath and imagine your own cells and your own spirit giving you a thumbs up.

Remove:

- I deserve to be in pain.
- I don't know how to live without pain.
- Pain is important to me.
- Pain is an important excuse for me.
- Pain serves me.
- I need pain in my life.
- I cannot learn without pain.

Replace with:

- I know how to live without pain.
- I deserve to live life pain-free.
- I know how to live life without using pain as an excuse.
- I am ready to release my need for pain.
- I release my need for pain.
- I can easily learn from a place of joy instead of pain.

Scribbling Page

Scribbling Page

DAY 24

Today we're working on beliefs around **passive aggression**. Feel free to write any thoughts you have about your experiences in the margins, or use the white space on this page to scribble out any emotions that come up as you do your tapping, removal, and replacement.

As a reminder: Tap while repeating aloud the belief you need to release. You may need to repeat the belief aloud several times. Imagine the old belief written out on a ribbon in your brain. As you tap and speak the belief, imagine the ribbon being sucked out of your head. Replace the old belief with a new belief by imagining the words of the new belief on a new, clean, bright ribbon. Tap while repeating the words of the new belief. Imagine the new belief ribbon threading into your brain and body and spirit. Imagine it wrapping around and in and through all of your individual cells. When you are done, take a deep breath and imagine your own cells and your own spirit giving you a thumbs up.

Remove:

- Passive aggression is an appropriate response.
- It is okay for me to be passive-aggressive.
- It is not okay for me to be direct about my feelings.
- I don't know how to live without passive aggression.
- Passive aggression keeps me safe.

Replace with:

- I know how to live without passive aggression.

- It can be safe for me to be clear about my feelings without being passive-aggressive.
- It is safe for me to be clear about my feelings without being passive-aggressive.
- I can be direct about my feelings.
- Passive aggression is an inappropriate behavior.

Scribbling Page

Scribbling Page

DAY 25

Today we're working on beliefs around **boundaries**. Feel free to write any thoughts you have about your experiences in the margins, or use the white space on this page to scribble out any emotions that come up as you do your tapping, removal, and replacement.

As a reminder: Tap while repeating aloud the belief you need to release. You may need to repeat the belief aloud several times. Imagine the old belief written out on a ribbon in your brain. As you tap and speak the belief, imagine the ribbon being sucked out of your head. Replace the old belief with a new belief by imagining the words of the new belief on a new, clean, bright ribbon. Tap while repeating the words of the new belief. Imagine the new belief ribbon threading into your brain and body and spirit. Imagine it wrapping around and in and through all of your individual cells. When you are done, take a deep breath and imagine your own cells and your own spirit giving you a thumbs up.

Remove:

- It is not safe for me to have clear boundaries.
- I don't know how to have boundaries.
- I should let other people into my space willy-nilly.
- I can't differentiate between my business and other people's business.
- I don't deserve strong boundaries.

Replace with:

- It is safe for me to have clear boundaries.
- I know God's divine definition of how to have clear boundaries.
- I know how to protect my space from other people's energies.
- I easily discern between what is my energy and my business, and what is other people's energy and other people's business.
- I deserve to have strong boundaries.

Scribbling Page

Scribbling Page

DAY 26

Today we're working on beliefs around **protection**. Feel free to write any thoughts you have about your experiences in the margins, or use the white space on this page to scribble out any emotions that come up as you do your tapping, removal, and replacement.

As a reminder: Tap while repeating aloud the belief you need to release. You may need to repeat the belief aloud several times. Imagine the old belief written out on a ribbon in your brain. As you tap and speak the belief, imagine the ribbon being sucked out of your head. Replace the old belief with a new belief by imagining the words of the new belief on a new, clean, bright ribbon. Tap while repeating the words of the new belief. Imagine the new belief ribbon threading into your brain and body and spirit. Imagine it wrapping around and in and through all of your individual cells. When you are done, take a deep breath and imagine your own cells and your own spirit giving you a thumbs up.

Remove:

- I don't deserve to be protected.
- I should be hurt.
- I am not worth protecting.
- Other people deserve protection more than me.
- There is not enough divine protection to go around.

Replace with:

- I DESERVE to be protected!
- I know how to live without needing to be hurt.

- I am worth protecting.
- I deserve protection as much as anyone else, and as much as EVERYONE else.
- There is more than enough divine protection to protect me and everyone else I care about.

Scribbling Page

Scribbling Page

DAY 27

Today we're working on beliefs around **hurt**. Feel free to write any thoughts you have about your experiences in the margins, or use the white space on this page to scribble out any emotions that come up as you do your tapping, removal, and replacement.

As a reminder: Tap while repeating aloud the belief you need to release. You may need to repeat the belief aloud several times. Imagine the old belief written out on a ribbon in your brain. As you tap and speak the belief, imagine the ribbon being sucked out of your head. Replace the old belief with a new belief by imagining the words of the new belief on a new, clean, bright ribbon. Tap while repeating the words of the new belief. Imagine the new belief ribbon threading into your brain and body and spirit. Imagine it wrapping around and in and through all of your individual cells. When you are done, take a deep breath and imagine your own cells and your own spirit giving you a thumbs up.

Remove:

- I deserve to be hurt.
- I am not a kind person.
- If others don't hurt me, I should hurt myself.
- I don't know how to live without being hurt.
- Being hurt makes me important.

Replace with:

- I deserve to be free from pain.

- I am a kind person.
- I know how to live without feeling I deserve to be hurt.
- I know how to live without being hurt.
- I am important without needing to be hurt.

Scribbling Page

Scribbling Page

DAY 28

Today we are working on beliefs about **sorrow**. Feel free to write any thoughts you have about your experiences in the margins, or use the white space on this page to scribble out any emotions that come up as you do your tapping, removal, and replacement.

As a reminder: Tap while repeating aloud the belief you need to release. You may need to repeat the belief aloud several times. Imagine the old belief written out on a ribbon in your brain. As you tap and speak the belief, imagine the ribbon being sucked out of your head. Replace the old belief with a new belief by imagining the words of the new belief on a new, clean, bright ribbon. Tap while repeating the words of the new belief. Imagine the new belief ribbon threading into your brain and body and spirit. Imagine it wrapping around and in and through all of your individual cells. When you are done, take a deep breath and imagine your own cells and your own spirit giving you a thumbs up.

Remove:

- Sorrow gives life meaning.
- It is important to feel sorrow often.
- I don't know how to live life without sorrow.
- My family brings me sorrow.
- Life should be sorrowful.
- Feeling sorrow means I'm taking sad things seriously.

Replace with:

- I know how to live life without sorrow.
- I am ready to release my sorrow.
- It is safe to turn my sorrows over to the Divine.
- I know how to take sad things seriously without drowning in the sorrow of it.
- It is important to find joy even in sorrowful times.

Scribbling Page

Scribbling Page

DAY 29

Today we are working on beliefs about **your healing journey**. Feel free to write any thoughts you have about your experiences in the margins, or use the white space on this page to scribble out any emotions that come up as you do your tapping, removal, and replacement.

As a reminder: Tap while repeating aloud the belief you need to release. You may need to repeat the belief aloud several times. Imagine the old belief written out on a ribbon in your brain. As you tap and speak the belief, imagine the ribbon being sucked out of your head. Replace the old belief with a new belief by imagining the words of the new belief on a new, clean, bright ribbon. Tap while repeating the words of the new belief. Imagine the new belief ribbon threading into your brain and body and spirit. Imagine it wrapping around and in and through all of your individual cells. When you are done, take a deep breath and imagine your own cells and your own spirit giving you a thumbs up.

Remove:

- I am scared to take the next steps on my healing journey.
- I don't deserve to heal.
- I don't know what to do next on my healing journey.
- I am not important enough to prioritize my own healing.
- Other people's healing is more important than my own.

Replace with:

- On a soul level, I know what to do next on my healing journey.
- I deserve healing.
- I deserve healing as much as anyone and everyone else.
- I know how to move forward fearlessly toward my healing.
- My healing is vastly important and worth prioritizing.

Scribbling Page

Scribbling Page

DAY 30

Today we are continuing to work on **your healing journey!** Feel free to write any thoughts you have about your experiences in the margins, or use the white space on this page to scribble out any emotions that come up as you do your tapping, removal, and replacement.

As a reminder: Tap while repeating aloud the belief you need to release. You may need to repeat the belief aloud several times. Imagine the old belief written out on a ribbon in your brain. As you tap and speak the belief, imagine the ribbon being sucked out of your head. Replace the old belief with a new belief by imagining the words of the new belief on a new, clean, bright ribbon. Tap while repeating the words of the new belief. Imagine the new belief ribbon threading into your brain and body and spirit. Imagine it wrapping around and in and through all of your individual cells. When you are done, take a deep breath and imagine your own cells and your own spirit giving you a thumbs up.

Remove:

- I don't know how to heal.
- Past healing attempts have failed me.
- My healing is doomed for failure.
- I don't know how to feel successful as I heal myself.
- I don't know how to recognize the positive changes in myself.

Replace with:

- I know how to recognize the positive changes in myself.
- I know how to heal.
- I can heal in the future and present even if past healing attempts have not gone well.
- My healing is destined for SUCCESS!
- I know how to feel successful as I heal myself!

Scribbling Page

Scribbling Page

CONCLUSION

YOU MADE IT! You did it! Congratulations! Thirty days of belief work! This is no small feat, and I am proud of you. Good work! I hope you are proud of yourself, too!

When I first started doing belief work, I didn't see big differences in myself right away. If you don't feel radically different, that's okay. That's normal. But pay attention to yourself, and to how you think and how you act. I would bet that as the days go on, you'll notice more and more how this daily habit of belief work has blessed your life.

You'll notice it in the little things, perhaps. You'll find yourself thinking in new ways. Perhaps it will be subtle, or perhaps you'll feel it in a bigger way. But the important thing is that **you have taken these steps on your healing journey.**

Every false or unhelpful belief we have floating around in our brains just causes problems. Clearing them out, even just a few at a time, adds up to create a big difference in the long term. In my opinion, you should feel very proud of yourself for this excellent work you have done in working to heal your unhelpful beliefs every day.

I invite you now to take some time to assess the changes you've noticed in yourself over the course of the past thirty days.

What changes have you noticed in how you think?

What changes have you noticed in your behavior?

What changes have you noticed in your reactions to others?

What is different about how you perceive the world now, as compared to before you began this belief work journey?

I invite you to really sit with these questions, to really take the time to ponder them. If you don't have the time, just asking these questions to yourself aloud a few times will get your mind working on the answers for you. You may be surprised at what insights come to you over the coming days as you open your mind to notice the changes that have developed in yourself over time.

When you are ready for the next step on your healing journey, I hope you do find me at allieduzettclasses.com. There are a number of free classes and group sessions there to help you get started, and I couldn't be more excited for you to continue the journey you've started here with this book.

Sending you love and light!

Allie Duzett
allie@allieduzett.com

Additional Resources From Allie Duzett

I work as a medical intuitive, and I do take on limited amounts of personal sessions. You can schedule a session at allieduzett.com/sessions.

I highly recommend getting on my email list at allieduzett.com. I send regular emails to those on my list with new sessions and lessons.

Allieduzettclasses.com is the hub for all my classes and group sessions. This is where I host numerous by-donation classes and lessons, including a robust Free Offerings session for those who need serious healing but don't have tons of cash to spend on it.

I have several other books available on Amazon, including *Deep Past Resolution* and *The Scribbling Solution. Deep Past Resolution* is about healing from pre-birth trauma, and *The Scribbling Solution* teaches the simplest, easiest technique I have discovered for healing very deep trauma.

Appendix: The Scribbling Technique

I have a video explanation of how to do this form of trauma release at allieduzett.com/scribbling. This is the primary exercise I teach my students in my official Deep Past Resolution online class.

All you need is paper and a pen. Actually, you don't even need a pen: the last time I did this exercise, it was with my finger on the screen of my phone. I have also simply used my hand in the air. A blunt crayon and a scrap paper work as well. Once you understand the concept, you can make this exercise work for you in many different contexts.

It is so easy.

The first step is to **identify what it is you're trying to work out**. Hopefully you already have a list of some items in your life you want to try scribbling out. And that's great! But if you don't, that's fine too.

When it comes to Deep Past trauma, limiting belief programming, or even the regular everyday bothers we experience in life, a lot of times we don't know the whole backstory… and sometimes we don't even know what exact emotions or struggles we're trying to clear. That's okay.

For example, you might not know the exact name of the feeling you feel when you think about a certain situation… and that's fine. It's enough to say, "I want to work on the feelings I feel when I think about X." That is good enough!

Label the top of your paper with whatever it is you're working on, as vaguely or as specifically as you can or want to. If you're dealing with anxiety about a weight issue, for example, you might label your paper "Fat" or "Betrayal of Body" or "Anger with Body." You might feel drawn to just label the paper with a specific weight, such as "182 lbs." If it's a limiting belief around your career, you might label it "Unhelpful Belief Affecting My Career" or "What will I do next?" or "What am I even doing with my life?"

However you feel you should label your paper, label your paper--as vaguely or specifically as you need to.

Step two is to imagine all the energy of the negative thing you're trying to clear as a specific color. I usually see mine as dark gray. Imagine all of that color gathering together throughout your body, and queuing up in the hand you'll be using.

And then:

SCRIBBLE!!!

Let your conscious mind take a break: it's not invited to this party. This is your subconscious mind's time to take over. Imagine the color of the negativity you're releasing going through your hand, into the writing utensil, and then out onto the paper (or even the screen of your phone, if you're scribbling with your finger on the screen).

If you're having trouble just letting your hand do its thing, then switch hands and let your non-dominant hand do the drawing.

The point is to let your body feel and release the emotion in a safe (but possibly intense!) way.

You may be surprised at how your hand and even your arm seems to take on a life of its own. That's what always shocks me, even though I know it will happen. I've done this exercise countless times, but it's still always such a surprise.

Keep going until your hand *spontaneously* makes **one single horizontal 0 shape**, a zero on its side, over and over again, right on top of itself. When you try to force your hand to scribble, it should naturally come back to making the empty hole shape. It is a shape symbolic of emptiness. If your ending horizontal 0 shape ends up filled in, or creating many loops that fill each other in, you are not done. You know you are done when no matter how you try to scribble on that issue, your hand naturally comes back to the empty horizontal oval.

Here's an experience that I had with this exercise once: I could feel a weird turbulence in my emotions and I didn't know what it was. So I grabbed a scrap paper and a blunt crayon, and told my hand to have at it. At first it I scribbled back and forth to the left, but then it got crazier and crazier until it was a dark blob on the lower right side of the scribble mass. The scribble ended with figure-8-type loops underneath that.

Next, I felt like asking myself, "Is there an energy that I need to heal this issue?" I didn't know what they meant, but I wrote down some numbers that felt right. You can ask yourself what "energies" you need to heal the emotional turbulence you are working to clear, and just write down whatever comes to you: numbers, names, flowers, ideas, whatever. Draw, color, write whatever comes to mind as something that will heal the issue.

You will find as you experiment with this technique that many things can happen--and you can feel very different afterwards. Even if what comes up during the exercise doesn't make sense.

Going back to my example, at that point, I felt like I could finally ask what the emotion was. The sense I felt in my heart was "self-resentment." I asked what I was resenting about myself, and got no answer. Later, I realized it was because I no longer had that self-resentment--it had been all scribbled out!

Once again, when your scribble is done, **you will know it because your hand will spontaneously create horizontal 0 shapes**. This has been true for virtually all of my clients, regardless of their background or whether I told them about this ahead of time. So **keep scribbling until your hand spontaneously creates horizontal 0s**. You will know you are truly done when you actively try to scribble and your hand naturally goes back to making that 0 shape instead.

To me, that horizontal 0 shape is symbolic of emptiness: it's a void where that trauma was. I love getting to that point in this exercise because when my hand starts making that shape, and I try scribbling a different way and just go back to that shape, I feel so different and so much happier.

For extra goodness, you can imagine filling up that empty 0 shape with light, symbolic of your own healing and choice to fill spaces with light that used to be full of trauma.

You will most likely want to throw away the paper when you are done with it, also. Typically, my used scribble papers have a very dark feeling to them. Often, it is worth it to me to pinch them by their corner and walk outside to throw them in the outside trash, and then come in and wash my hands.

I wrote earlier that you can actually do this exercise on your phone. One of my students discovered this when she tried it out on a scribbling app she'd gotten for one of her kids. If you do this exercise using your phone, afterwards, you will want to imagine light from the Divine coming down from the heavens and washing any residual darkness out of your phone!

When it comes to belief work, this exercise is fabulous because it takes something that can seem huge and intense, and allows us to eradicate it without muscle testing, without fancy magnets, without really anything. You don't need to be properly polarized or grounded to clear trauma this way--you don't even need to be sure what the trauma is. You just choose what you want to work on and get started.

One precaution with this exercise is to possibly be mindful of the magnitude of what you seek to use it for. **Very large traumas may be too much to try scribbling out all at once.** And once you start scribbling, you don't want to stop until you've gotten that horizontal 0 shape.

So it can be wise to *set the intention ahead of time that the trauma you wish to work on will be separated into smaller pieces that can be scribbled out in five-minute increments.* **I like to imagine the trauma I am working with, and then imagine smashing it with a hammer into smaller pieces that are more manageable to scribble out.**

This exercise sounds very easy when you read about it, but after a few minutes your arm can really get tired! So it's good to break down the trauma you want to clear into smaller pieces before you commit to scribbling it out all the way.

A story comes to mind of one client in particular who was a victim of extreme abuse as a child. When she attempted to scribble on it, she did not break down the traumas into smaller pieces first and ended up scribbling for many, many minutes, completely destroying many sheets of paper--scribbling right through the papers--and still did not find resolution.

When you are working with a trauma that is large, often you want to break it down first by imagining it breaking into smaller pieces, and then work on it one piece at a time until it is resolved.

It's like eating an elephant. How do you eat an elephant? One bite at a time.

How do you resolve and release all the traumas, blocks, and resistances holding you back? One five-minute increment of work at a time. Over time, those five-minute investments in your health and wellness will really pay off. It's the law of compound interest!

If you get started scribbling not realizing how big of an energy something is, you can at that time mentally chop off that energy into a smaller piece and set the intention that you will finish scribbling out this portion of energy now. That is an easy way to fix things if you accidentally "bite off more than you can chew" with this work.

Analyzing Your Scribbles

One question I get fairly regularly about this exercise is if the shapes you scribble mean anything. My opinion is that they must, but I have no idea what the shapes mean, and it feels extremely unimportant to me to analyze them.

To me, the important thing here is using the technique to release and resolve trauma without needing to dig into lots of pesky details.

The beauty of scribbling as a release technique is **how much you DON'T need to know**. The point of scribbling is to release negative energies without the hassle of grounding, polarizing, muscle testing, and anything else.

To me, analyzing scribbles after the fact just adds an unnecessary complication to the work. So, I say: don't bother with that, it's a waste of time. You could use those five minutes you're analyzing your scribble to just scribble something else out! To me personally, that is a better use of time.

If you feel inspired to psychoanalyze your scribbles, that is fine with me--just know that I will be unlikely to offer additional wisdom about their meaning!

To me, the only meaning of a scribble that matters is: what was once in, is now OUT!

HOORAY!

For more on how to use scribbling for anxiety, depression, weight loss, relationships, and manifestation, please order the book The Scribbling Solution on Amazon.com.

Printed in Great Britain
by Amazon

33643760R00086